KEEP FIT TRACKER
Fitness, Nutrition, and Mindset:
Your All-in-One Wellness Tracker

2021 LeadHer Publishing

Copyright© 2021 Jeenie Brasseur/LeadHer Publishing

All rights reserved. No part of this book may be reproduced, scanned, or distributed in any printed or electronic form without permission. No portion of this book may be used in any alternative manner whatsoever without express written consent from the publisher LeadHer Publishing.

The author of this book has made every effort to ensure the accuracy of the information they have provided at the time of publication. The author does not assume and hereby disclaims any liability to any party for loss, damage, or disruption caused by errors of omissions, whether such errors or omissions were from accident, negligence, or any other cause. This book is not a replacement for medical advice from a registered physician. The author has independently contributed to the content of this book, irrespective of the publisher's contributions, viewpoints, or advice.

The publisher is not responsible for websites, social media, or other content that is not owned by the publisher.

Cover Design - Kristie Verdurmen
Interior Design - Christina Williams
ISBN: 978-1-990352-03-4

For more information on the author, visit www.keepfitwomen.com
instagram.com/keepfit.women
instagram.com/jeeniesjourney

For more information on the publisher, visit www.lead-her.com
instagram.com/leadherpublishing
or email admin@lead-her.com

FITNESS, NUTRITION AND MINDSET: YOUR ALL-IN-ONE WELLNESS TRACKER

KEEP FIT *tracker*

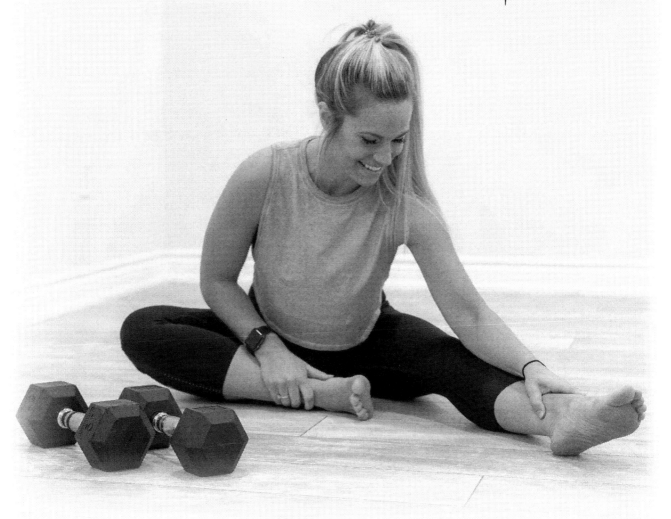

JEENIE BRASSEUR

Introduction

Hey friend. *Waves* Are you ready to set your fitness and health goals, stay on track, and keep insanely motivated along the way? Good, 'cause I'm ready to help you!

Getting your workouts in, eating well, and being mindful are all *awesome*. I commend you on striving to be your best! What's even better, though, is that when you actually track your habits, you can get a visible and tangible representation of the progress you're making. Seeing progress is a key factor in keeping you motivated to move your body, reach for optimal foods, and practice mindfulness daily. By tracking your habits you will be able to witness both quick and long-term wins that will keep you on the path to a balanced, fit, and healthy lifestyle.

Progress is so much more than just noticeable changes in your external body composition. Progress can be consistency over time. Progress can be achieving a certain length of workout. Progress can be becoming aware of how you feel after consuming certain foods. Progress can be noticing that you are more calm and present throughout the day. These pages are designed to keep you on track, accountable, and motivated to reach whatever goal you set for yourself.

Here's the deal: I designed this workbook to be a companion to your desire to build a fit and healthy lifestyle. Inside, you'll see that there are three sections that align closely with the physical representation of KeepFit Women's four integral pillars. (The fourth pillar is COMMUNITY, so make sure you're finding us online so that you can see the difference that a strong community can make in your success!).

FITNESS, NUTRITION, and MINDSET are the other three pillars in our approach to healthy living. This journal has a section for each pillar, so that you can hold yourself accountable to connecting with all three pieces.

You may complete one page from each section every day. On other days, you may just use the nutrition and mindset sections, because I understand and respect that you will likely not be doing a workout every single day. (In fact, I don't encourage anyone to workout seven days a week, as it's much more difficult to maintain and isn't as sustainable as committing to 2-4 workouts each week. Ultimately, it will be up to you, but I didn't want you to assume that you're meant to fill out a fitness tracker page every day!)

The fitness tracker will allow you to track your metrics for any type of workout that you complete. Whether you're focusing on strength, cardiovascular endurance, flexibility, or a particular style of workout, you can keep track of your progress here.

The nutrition tracker will hold you accountable for making smart meal decisions *for your body*, and observing things like hunger cues and how you feel after you eat specific foods. Everyone's body responds in different ways to the food we eat, and I encourage you to become more mindful about what you're eating, when, and what quality of foods you're putting into your body.

The mindset tracker will help you focus on specific things so that you can adjust and fine tune the way you're noticing the world. The mindset tracker can be completed every day, and I encourage you to do just that. Mindset work is often taken one of two ways: it's either too simple — so we assume that it couldn't possibly impact change — or it's "too much work" to fill in some mindfulness questions each day. In either case, it's common to ditch the practice altogether, so then we're not even giving it a fighting chance to make a difference. I encourage you to challenge whatever existing beliefs you have about mindset work and commit to doing one page every day until you complete the journal.

Just like many tools we have access to in life, this journal is meant to support you along your journey to keeping fit — whatever that looks like for you. I challenge you to take it seriously, commit to completing all of the pages inside the book, and then see how you feel after you've done just that. This journal will become a tangible example of your accountability and commitment, and in turn has the power to transform competence into confidence. With each workout, healthy meal, and by granting yourself time to focus on yourself and your mind, you're putting in the necessary work to establish a strong foundation on which you can operate your entire life.

So, the question is: Will you start?

I can't wait to see how you commit to yourself. You are the most important person in your life. Make sure you're putting yourself first so that you can feel your best when you interact with others important to you.

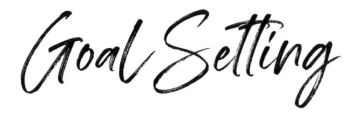

Goal Setting

Before you begin your journey of daily/weekly tracking, it may be helpful to think about what your fitness and health related goals are for the next 3-6 months. I'm not just talking about weight loss here. You may have that in mind, but I encourage you to consider other success markers to keep at the forefront of your mind along the way. There are so many incredible ways that you can progress toward your goals, and I challenge you to think outside the box and reach for something that's not just related to your external appearance.

Do you want to increase the amount of weight you lift? Do you want to feel less bloated? Do you want to be able to do a full push up on your toes without struggling or sacrificing form? Do you want to feel more joyful each day? Do you want to create consistent healthy habits that you *finally* stick to? Do you want to learn how to do a pull-up and execute a few unassisted? Do you want to feel better, inside and out, body and mind?

Think about some things you'd like to work on over the next few months, and note them here. Come back to this often to check in on how you're progressing.

YOUR GOALS

Goal 1:

Goal 2:

Goal 3:

HOW TO USE THIS TRACKER:

Okay, so... how do I actually use this tracker? Great question! I've given an example of each page at the start of each section, in case you've never used something like this to track your habits. The idea is quite simple: When you complete a workout, write down the details on one of the fitness pages. As you navigate your healthy eating strategy, log your meals on one of the nutrition pages. Each day, complete one of the mindset pages during a time in your day when you have a few minutes to connect with yourself more deeply, reflect, and journal. Ultimately, though, you can use this journal however you see fit.

If you have experience tracking your workouts or journaling in some way, then this process will be no sweat (pun intended)! I want you to be able to organize your workouts, track your progress, keep accountable to your desire to eat whole, nutritious food, set and monitor your goals, and make changes to your mindset with regular focus and gratitude. I also want you to be able to take this little book with you anywhere you go; drop it in your purse, keep it in your gym bag, and pack it with you if you travel. Keep it close, keep it handy, and keep focused on the ways you want to *keep fit*. Little by little, we'll get there together!

I'll show you the fitness section first, and explain how to best use those pages. Then you'll see loads of space for you to fill in with your workouts. The next section will be nutrition, and then mindset; and I'll gxive you an idea of how to incorporate those pages, too.

Ready!?

Jeenie's Journey

I have a vivid memory of being eight years old and casually gliding up to a soccer field. The soccer field was a place where I felt safe and truly joyful. I loved every aspect of the sport. I would strut my way up the field, sit on the fragrant, freshly cut grass, put on my cleats, tighten my pony tail, and await kick off with a whole body buzz of anticipation. I was always excited to be in the mental and physical zone where I felt strong, capable, and like a badass in my own body. At the tender age of eight, I didn't realize what an incredibly powerful and impactful feeling it was to have default positive feelings about my body, and what it could do for me through the execution of physical activities like sports. I had no concept of the way that this feeling would impact my body image. I had no sense of the beautiful and positive foundation that I was building for myself in future years. I was unaware, and just blissfully basked in all of those good feelings.

I grew up not only playing competitive soccer, but I also played hockey and pursued a job as a snowboard instructor. I dabbled in volleyball, basketball, running, and even curling. I guess you could say I was quite the aspiring athlete.

Years passed, and my commitment and love for sports continued. When I received my acceptance letter to attend the University of Waterloo for their Recreation Therapy program, I immediately emailed the women's varsity soccer coach. I desperately wanted to be a part of the team. The idea of trying out on a new team, with new coaches and a heightened level of competition was intimidating, but I had my eyes on a goal and I went for it. After months of sprint training, lifting weights, long runs, and hours on the soccer field practicing by myself, I was invited onto the pitch to showcase my skills. I was definitely not the most talented player (by a long shot) but the coach saw my grit, determination, and passion for the sport.

After two weeks of gruelling tryouts, cuts were made to the team roster. Much to my excitement, I made the team. I went on to spend the next four years (from 2008 to 2012) playing for the University of Waterloo Women's

Soccer team. I was never the best player on the team, but I can say with confidence that I trained hard and earned my spot on that field. Over these years as a competitive athlete, I had the opportunity to informally train many women on my team, and some of my fellow students and friends, too. I would create workout outlines and lead my team members through the workouts that I created. I remember feeling completely in the zone as I led these workouts. It was an incredibly joyous time in my life. Unbeknownst to me at that time, this opportunity allowed me to combine my love for sport, physical activity, and empowering others through coaching these women to feel good about what their bodies could *do*, not just what their bodies *looked like*. Some of my absolute best memories from my twenties were spent on the soccer pitch, with bloodied and blistered feet, sore muscles, and a keen mental awareness that my body was a tool that I could adjust and enhance to compete.

All of these experiences with sport in my childhood and throughout my 20s had such an impact on my life, specifically my perception of my body and overall self-image. I truly saw my body as this amazing tool designed to support me, carry me, and help me pursue the things that I wanted to go after in my life — on and off the proverbial "pitch."

I learned through my experiences with sport that if I was willing to put the work in and train hard, I could achieve the physical results that I wanted. Nobody is born an expert — and I most certainly wasn't an expert at soccer or any other sport — but I was determined to chase after the goals I desired. I learned that I couldn't control skill or talent, but I could control the effort I put into improving, growing, and developing. My body was so much more than how it looked in a bathing suit or a pretty dress. I felt really strong and powerful in my own skin. I was fortunate to almost always feel confident in my clothes, and if I didn't, I knew how to train to not only get "in shape" from an athletic perspective, but to also get the physical body composition that I wanted.

This all came crashing down in 2013.

After I graduated from University in 2012, I saved every single penny I could for more than a year. I took this money and (much to my parents' dismay) bought a one-way ticket to South America. I was going to travel across South America, Southeast Asia, and Australia, and I was going to do it largely by myself. I had this grand vision of the backpacking adventure to come, and once again, I had my eyes on a goal and I went for it.

I spent the next year traveling around the world, making my way from hostel to hostel. I met incredible people from all over the world and had countless (and priceless) adventures along the way. I spent most of my time seeking said adventure; jogging through Bangkok, doing yoga on the beach in Vietnam, hiking my way to the top of Machu Picchu, learning to surf in Ecuador, climbing the stairs to ancient temples in Cambodia, swimming in open water with sharks in the Galapagos Islands… It was a thrilling time, to say the least. But during this year when I was traveling, something started to feel a bit off in my physical body.

During the time that I was traveling, I had started to gain weight despite keeping relatively active. I started to notice that I was constantly tired. I remember deciding to go to bed early instead of attending a midnight beach party on an island in Thailand, which my close friends would know was not like me. Something just started to feel off. My sex drive had nosedived to zero. Then, the biggest red flag appeared: I stopped menstruating. By the time I landed in Australia in late 2013, I hadn't had a period in over four months. I was anxious to know what was going on with my body, so as soon as I landed in Australia I contacted a doctor for an appointment. I desperately tried to explain that something was wrong. To my disappointment, I was essentially told that "gaining weight around the age of 25 is normal" and to wait and come back in a few months if I still hadn't resumed a normal menstrual cycle.

I cannot even count how many doctor appointments I had, nor how many tests I went through to pinpoint what exactly was going on. I would leave each visit so disheartened. I was never given an explanation as to why my body looked and felt so different, despite continuing to live a healthy lifestyle. I had changed nothing in my lifestyle, diet, or movement behaviours, yet my body was changing and holding onto weight without any explanation.

It was during these months of sheer frustration and hopelessness that I started to obsess over exercise and nutrition. For the first time in my life, I could not control how my body looked and felt. I had gained about 40 extra pounds at this point. Being only 5'1", this excess weight was very noticeable and suddenly my clothes weren't fitting. All of the training techniques and nutrition approaches I had learned over the years in sport suddenly had no effect. I felt lost and confused. What had happened? I started counting calories, which was something I had never even considered before. I did countless hours of researching "the best way" to exercise for the sole purpose of losing weight. I read nutrition blogs constantly, I watched YouTube videos, I even tried following a strict bodybuilding workout program. After months of hard work, strict nutrition, keeping laser focused on "staying on track," and working out more often with higher intensity — the scale hadn't budged at all, I was still exhausted, and I had still not had a period.

I remember catching a glimpse of my reflection in a store window one day while on a walk in the streets of Sydney, and I literally didn't recognize myself. The reflection staring back at me was so much larger than I was accustomed to seeing. I felt defeated. My body had changed so much, both inside and out. I felt like an absolute stranger in my own body. I began to lose that sense of innate wisdom that I had developed from such an early age; that wisdom that I had grown to rely on in regard to my body. I started to question if I really knew my body as well as I had thought. I began to question my identity as a "fitness lover" because I felt that I no longer looked like one. I simply started to lose hope that I would ever feel like myself, the keeper of this beautiful and strong tool, again.

Approximately six months after my initial appointment, my team of doctors began doing extensive testing and discovered that I had some sort of hormone imbalance. I did my best to explain that this body, this 40 pound heavier body, was not normal for me. I remember trying to explain that I knew fitness, I knew healthy eating, and it wasn't working. Something was wrong and I felt like no one was listening. At each appointment I would enter the doctor's office hopeful, thinking that perhaps they had found a reason for my changing body, and each time I would exit, in tears, being told to come back in a couple of months for more testing. Each time, I felt a heaviness in my heart and a sense of hopelessness.

It was during months of blood tests, external ultrasounds, internal ultrasounds, biopsies, and brain scans that I started to realize that this approach to fitness — a strict and rigid method — wasn't serving me mentally. It was adding stress to my life and sabotaging the beautiful relationship that I had built with my body and body image. My body was still a wonderful tool and symbol of strength, but maybe, just maybe, I needed to focus on health throughout my whole body and not just from a perspective in which my goals were simply to change the composition and external appearance of my body.

Over time, it dawned on me: What if I adjusted my approach? What if I started taking care of my WHOLE self? What if I approach fitness from a whole body-health perspective? I mean, at this point, what did I have to lose? I slowly realized that being a "fitness lover" did not have anything to do with how I *looked*, but everything to do with how I approached fitness, led my life, and how I desired to lead others along the way, too.

I shifted away from strict calorie counting, and started to integrate nutritious (but high calorie) foods, like high fat avocados, again.

I started adding yoga to my routine, instead of just weightlifting and high intensity training.

I started to journal my experiences.

I started taking note of how I felt inside (not just how I looked on the outside).

I started to slowly view my body as a powerful tool again.

And of course, I continued to tirelessly advocate for myself at each doctor's appointment.

By the end of 2015, I had moved home to Canada and slowly began to regulate my hormone functions again. The problem with something as intangible as a hormone imbalance is that I cannot tell you exactly what suddenly resolved the issues. In the same way that none of the doctors could figure out *exactly* what was going on beneath the surface, nobody ever gave me a full-on diagnosis or protocol to 'correct' the issues I was having. In fact, hardly any of the doctors I visited even believed what I was trying to convey. At 40 pounds over my typical and normal body weight, I wasn't exactly what they would have diagnosed as "overweight." It was overweight for *me* and *my* body (and it didn't make sense that I couldn't manipulate it through diet and exercise), but I wasn't officially diagnosed at any clinical level of weight gain, so most of the doctors didn't take my concerns seriously.

I also don't know exactly what the "cure" was, or how my hormones started to balance again after a year of intense and rapid body changes. I started removing the restrictions I had set for myself. I started listening more intuitively to my body, my desires, and my need for rest and recovery, but I was never given an exact protocol to observe in order to "fix" myself. But what I can tell you is that I learned an insane amount about my willingness to advocate for myself and dig deeper to try to figure out what was going on, and this is something I still encourage any of the women I work with inside my fitness and coaching programs to do.

I had dramatically evolved in the process of this experience, and even though I can't say for certain what it was or how I managed to get back to some sense of normalcy, I have made it my mission to support women on their health journeys so that they can learn how to intuitively pay attention to their own version of normal, and feel supported as they attempt to maintain or adjust their own body composition, body image, and confidence levels.

I know what it's like to feel unsuccessful at achieving the results you're hoping for, and in most cases, I have the tools, resources, and knowledge to be able to support women without any major contraindications on how they can best support themselves in their pursuit of living a healthy lifestyle. I am not a hormone expert — nor will I ever claim to be — but I know my experiences in battling undiagnosed body issues have trained me well for helping women learn more about their bodies and how to know when something is "off" that requires further investigation.

From an early age, I had the experience of viewing my body as a tool. Now I *also* have gained a deeper understanding of fitness, nutrition, and **mindset.** I know how important it is to integrate a balanced and sustainable approach to fitness and nutrition outside of what your external body looks like.

I've always been interested in movement, exercise, fitness, nutrition, and health. First, so that my body could perform for me via sport as a child and young adult, and then later, so that I could operate at my best and comfortably sustain the adventurous lifestyle that I wanted to maintain. As I ventured into the next stage of my life, I knew I wanted to help support others in their own health journeys so that they could have someone to lean on during the times they felt uncertain, unclear, or unsure of the next best step for their own unique circumstances.

I had spent years informally training my friends and giving people fitness and nutrition advice on my social media account. But it was on a rainy Wednesday afternoon in September 2015 that I returned home from a soccer-inspired workout while just about five months pregnant with my daughter, Jaelyn, and I had an epiphany. I wanted to continue guiding and training women, but I wanted to make it official. I wanted to create a community where I could help keep women fit and healthy — whatever that looked like for them. I wanted to show women how to love their bodies, no matter what size or shape, for the way their bodies can support them in life and in health. I wanted to help women understand that their health is their responsibility, but that they aren't alone in their pursuit of a healthier lifestyle. I wanted to help keep women fit. I set my mind to a goal, and once again, I went for it. While pregnant, I took several personal training and nutrition courses, and just weeks before my daughter was born I officially launched *KeepFit Women*.

I am so passionate about this work. I am so keen to help women understand their own bodies, their own health, their own version of "fit"... and I don't plan on stopping any time soon. If you haven't yet, I encourage you to find me on social media and connect with me and the KeepFit Women Community. The level of support inside this community is higher than I ever dreamed of, and I'm so excited and honoured that I get to support women inside this space on a daily basis.

Keeping fit is so much more than just what your body may look like on the outside. I am committed to helping women understand this, and I'm here for **you** if you need help to see it this way, too.

A NOTE ON COMMUNITY

Intrinsic motivation and work ethic can only get you so far. I speak from experience when I say that being surrounded by an incredible group of like-minded women can help propel you forward and give you that extra sense of accountability that you need to be successful in achieving your goals. If this is something that you hope to experience, or if you are feeling like you need that extra push, I invite you to connect with me and the Keep-Fit Women community on our social media platforms.

Tag me on social media and show me a photo of you using your tracker. I will be sure to personally send you a message of encouragement.

I absolutely cannot wait to connect with you and watch your journey unfold.

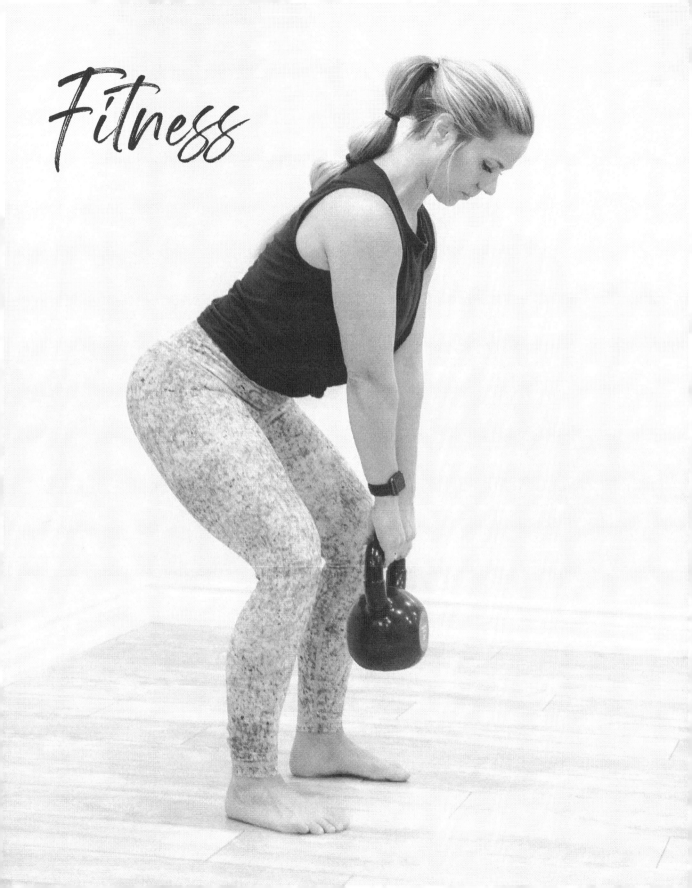

Movement

Why track your movement? Well, it's just like anything else in your life; energy flows where attention goes. Sure, you can still maintain a good movement schedule if you don't track it. But when you write down what you've done, it gives you tangible evidence of what you did, how you felt, and how you've improved after a certain period of time.

Writing things down is beneficial in so many ways. Movement is no exception. If you keep track of how you're committing to moving your body, it can help you solidify the habit and the practice of the thing you're tracking.

TIP: If you haven't worked out in a while (or ever!) don't set yourself up for failure by pledging to workout 7 days a week for 2 hours at a time. Start small. 2-3 workouts per week is more than enough for you to establish a routine and start feeling (first) and seeing (later) results. I'm far more concerned that you build a sustainable habit around fitness. Focusing on the habit will create long-term results that will last a lifetime!

If you've never tracked your workouts before, you may be a little unsure of what some of the columns mean. No problem! I've included an example page to show you how you might fill in your workouts.

TIP: You don't need to fill in every line every workout. I just wanted to ensure that you had enough space to do lots of movements, where applicable! If you have a particularly long workout with lots of different moves, you can always use two pages that day.

MOVEMENT

Workout plan/type: Leg day　　　　**Date:** July 30th

Length: 30 minutes　　**Focus:** Strength

movement	reps	sets	weight	time
Goblet squats	12	4	40lbs	-
Jumping jacks	-	-	bodyweight	1 min.
Sumo squats	12	3	40lbs	-
Squat jumps	-	-	bw	1 min.
Straight leg deadlifts	12	3	60lbs	-
Glute bridges	10	5	20lbs	-
Donkey kickbacks	15	3	bw	-
10 minute walk as a cool down				

[X] Post Workout STRETCH　　[X] Post Workout WATER

Something positive from today's workout

　　I really pushed myself and felt strong

How I feel after today's workout

　　Motivated and empowered

MOVEMENT

Workout plan/Type Date:

Length: [ ] Focus: [ ]

movement	reps	sets	weight	time

☐ Post Workout STRETCH   ☐ Post Workout WATER

Something positive from today's workout

How I feel after today's workout

MOVEMENT

Workout plan/type   Date:

Length: [   ]   Focus: [   ]

movement	reps	sets	weight	time

☐ Post Workout STRETCH   ☐ Post Workout WATER

Something positive from today's workout

How I feel after today's workout

MOVEMENT

Workout plan/type

Date:

Length: Focus:

movement	reps	sets	weight	time

☐ Post Workout STRETCH ☐ Post Workout WATER

Something positive from today's workout

How I feel after today's workout

MOVEMENT

Workout plan/type   Date:

Length: [   ]   Focus: [   ]

movement	reps	sets	weight	time

☐ Post Workout STRETCH   ☐ Post Workout WATER

Something positive from today's workout

How I feel after today's workout

MOVEMENT

Workout plan/Type   Date:

Length: [ ]   Focus: [ ]

movement	reps	sets	weight	time

☐ Post Workout STRETCH   ☐ Post Workout WATER

Something positive from today's workout

How I feel after today's workout

MOVEMENT

Workout plan/type   Date:

Length: [   ]   Focus: [   ]

movement	reps	sets	weight	time

☐ Post Workout STRETCH   ☐ Post Workout WATER

Something positive from today's workout

How I feel after today's workout

MOVEMENT

Workout plan/Type Date:

Length: _____   Focus: _____

movement	reps	sets	weight	time

☐ Post Workout STRETCH   ☐ Post Workout WATER

Something positive from today's workout

How I feel after today's workout

MOVEMENT

Workout plan/Type   Date:

Length: [   ]   Focus: [   ]

movement	reps	sets	weight	time

☐ Post Workout STRETCH   ☐ Post Workout WATER

Something positive from today's workout

How I feel after today's workout

MOVEMENT

Workout plan/type   Date:

Length: [ ]   Focus: [ ]

movement	reps	sets	weight	time

[ ] Post Workout STRETCH   [ ] Post Workout WATER

Something positive from today's workout

How I feel after today's workout

MOVEMENT

Workout plan/type Date:

Length: _____ Focus: _____

movement	reps	sets	weight	time

MOVEMENT

☐ Post Workout STRETCH   ☐ Post Workout WATER

Something positive from today's workout

How I feel after today's workout

MOVEMENT

Workout plan/Type Date:

Length: Focus:

movement	reps	sets	weight	time

☐ Post Workout STRETCH ☐ Post Workout WATER

Something positive from today's workout

How I feel after today's workout

MOVEMENT

Workout plan/type Date:

Length: Focus:

movement	reps	sets	weight	time

☐ Post Workout STRETCH ☐ Post Workout WATER

Something positive from today's workout

How I feel after today's workout

MOVEMENT

Workout plan/Type Date:

Length: [ ]   Focus: [ ]

movement	reps	sets	weight	time

☐ Post Workout STRETCH   ☐ Post Workout WATER

Something positive from today's workout

How I feel after today's workout

MOVEMENT

Workout plan/type Date:

Length: _____ Focus: _____

movement	reps	sets	weight	time

☐ Post Workout STRETCH ☐ Post Workout WATER

Something positive from today's workout

How I feel after today's workout

MOVEMENT

Workout plan/Type

Date:

Length: Focus:

movement	reps	sets	weight	time

☐ Post Workout STRETCH ☐ Post Workout WATER

Something positive from today's workout

How I feel after today's workout

MOVEMENT

Workout plan/Type   Date:

Length: [   ]   Focus: [   ]

movement	reps	sets	weight	time

☐ Post Workout STRETCH   ☐ Post Workout WATER

Something positive from today's workout

How I feel after today's workout

MOVEMENT

Workout plan/Type   Date:

Length: [ ]   Focus: [ ]

movement	reps	sets	weight	time

☐ Post Workout STRETCH   ☐ Post Workout WATER

Something positive from today's workout

How I feel after today's workout

MOVEMENT

Workout plan/type   Date:

Length: ☐   Focus: ☐

movement	reps	sets	weight	time

☐ Post Workout STRETCH   ☐ Post Workout WATER

Something positive from today's workout

How I feel after today's workout

MOVEMENT

Workout plan/Type   Date:

Length: [   ]   Focus: [   ]

movement	reps	sets	weight	time

☐ Post Workout STRETCH   ☐ Post Workout WATER

Something positive from today's workout

How I feel after today's workout

MOVEMENT

Workout plan/Type   Date:

Length: [ ]   Focus: [ ]

movement	reps	sets	weight	time

[ ] Post Workout STRETCH   [ ] Post Workout WATER

Something positive from today's workout

How I feel after today's workout

MOVEMENT

Workout plan/Type   Date:

Length: [   ]   Focus: [   ]

movement	reps	sets	weight	time

☐ Post Workout STRETCH   ☐ Post Workout WATER

Something positive from today's workout

How I feel after today's workout

MOVEMENT

Workout plan/type   Date:

Length: [ ]   Focus: [ ]

movement	reps	sets	weight	time

☐ Post Workout STRETCH   ☐ Post Workout WATER

Something positive from today's workout

How I feel after today's workout

MOVEMENT

Workout plan/Type Date:

Length: _____ Focus: _____

movement	reps	sets	weight	time

☐ Post Workout STRETCH ☐ Post Workout WATER

Something positive from today's workout

How I feel after today's workout

MOVEMENT

Workout plan/type Date:

Length: ____ Focus: ____

movement	reps	sets	weight	time

☐ Post Workout STRETCH   ☐ Post Workout WATER

Something positive from today's workout

How I feel after today's workout

MOVEMENT

Workout plan/Type   Date:

Length: _____   Focus: _____

movement	reps	sets	weight	time

☐ Post Workout STRETCH   ☐ Post Workout WATER

Something positive from today's workout

How I feel after today's workout

MOVEMENT

Workout plan/Type   Date:

Length: _____   Focus: _____

movement	reps	sets	weight	time

☐ Post Workout STRETCH   ☐ Post Workout WATER

Something positive from today's workout

How I feel after today's workout

MOVEMENT

Workout plan/Type Date:

Length: [ ]   Focus: [ ]

movement	reps	sets	weight	time

☐ Post Workout STRETCH   ☐ Post Workout WATER

Something positive from today's workout

How I feel after today's workout

MOVEMENT

Workout plan/Type Date:

Length: _____ Focus: _____

movement	reps	sets	weight	time

☐ Post Workout STRETCH   ☐ Post Workout WATER

Something positive from today's workout

How I feel after today's workout

MOVEMENT

Workout plan/Type　　　　　　　　　　　　　　Date:

Length: ☐　　　Focus: ☐

movement	reps	sets	weight	time

☐ Post Workout STRETCH　　☐ Post Workout WATER

Something positive from today's workout

How I feel after today's workout

MOVEMENT

Workout plan/type   Date:

Length: [　　　　　]   Focus: [　　　　　]

movement	reps	sets	weight	time

☐ Post Workout STRETCH   ☐ Post Workout WATER

Something positive from today's workout

How I feel after today's workout

MOVEMENT

Workout plan/Type   Date:

Length: [   ]   Focus: [   ]

movement	reps	sets	weight	time

☐ Post Workout STRETCH   ☐ Post Workout WATER

Something positive from today's workout

How I feel after today's workout

MOVEMENT

Workout plan/type   Date:

Length: [   ]   Focus: [   ]

movement	reps	sets	weight	time

☐ Post Workout STRETCH   ☐ Post Workout WATER

Something positive from today's workout

How I feel after today's workout

MOVEMENT

Workout plan/Type Date:

Length: _____ Focus: _____

movement	reps	sets	weight	time

☐ Post Workout STRETCH   ☐ Post Workout WATER

Something positive from today's workout

How I feel after today's workout

MOVEMENT

Workout plan/type   Date:

Length: [   ]   Focus: [   ]

movement	reps	sets	weight	time

☐ Post Workout STRETCH   ☐ Post Workout WATER

Something positive from today's workout

How I feel after today's workout

MOVEMENT

Workout plan/type   Date:

Length: [   ]   Focus: [   ]

movement	reps	sets	weight	time

☐ Post Workout STRETCH   ☐ Post Workout WATER

Something positive from today's workout

How I feel after today's workout

MOVEMENT

Workout plan/type   Date:

Length: [   ]   Focus: [   ]

movement	reps	sets	weight	time

☐ Post Workout STRETCH   ☐ Post Workout WATER

Something positive from today's workout

How I feel after today's workout

MOVEMENT

Workout plan/Type   Date:

Length: [ ]   Focus: [ ]

movement	reps	sets	weight	time

☐ Post Workout STRETCH   ☐ Post Workout WATER

Something positive from today's workout

How I feel after today's workout

MOVEMENT

Workout plan/Type   Date:

Length: [ ]   Focus: [ ]

movement	reps	sets	weight	time

☐ Post Workout STRETCH   ☐ Post Workout WATER

Something positive from today's workout

How I feel after today's workout

MOVEMENT

Workout plan/Type Date:

Length: _____   Focus: _____

movement	reps	sets	weight	time

☐ Post Workout STRETCH   ☐ Post Workout WATER

Something positive from today's workout

How I feel after today's workout

MOVEMENT

Workout plan/Type   Date:

Length: [ ]   Focus: [ ]

movement	reps	sets	weight	time

☐ Post Workout STRETCH   ☐ Post Workout WATER

Something positive from today's workout

How I feel after today's workout

MOVEMENT

Workout plan/type   Date:

Length: [ ]   Focus: [ ]

movement	reps	sets	weight	time

☐ Post Workout STRETCH   ☐ Post Workout WATER

Something positive from today's workout

How I feel after today's workout

MOVEMENT

Workout plan/type　　　　　　　　　　　　　　　Date:

Length: ☐　　　　　Focus: ☐

movement	reps	sets	weight	time

☐ Post Workout STRETCH　　　☐ Post Workout WATER

Something positive from today's workout

How I feel after today's workout

MOVEMENT

Workout plan/Type　　　　　　　　　　　　　　　Date:

Length: ☐　　　　　　Focus: ☐

movement	reps	sets	weight	time

☐ Post Workout STRETCH　　　☐ Post Workout WATER

Something positive from today's workout

How I feel after today's workout

MOVEMENT

Workout plan/Type: Date:

Length: [   ]   Focus: [   ]

movement	reps	sets	weight	time

☐ Post Workout STRETCH   ☐ Post Workout WATER

Something positive from today's workout

How I feel after today's workout

MOVEMENT

Workout plan/Type   Date:

Length: [ ]   Focus: [ ]

movement	reps	sets	weight	time

☐ Post Workout STRETCH   ☐ Post Workout WATER

Something positive from today's workout

How I feel after today's workout

MOVEMENT

Workout plan/Type Date:

Length: [   ]   Focus: [   ]

movement	reps	sets	weight	time

☐ Post Workout STRETCH   ☐ Post Workout WATER

Something positive from today's workout

How I feel after today's workout

MOVEMENT

Workout plan/Type Date:

Length: [ ] Focus: [ ]

movement	reps	sets	weight	time

☐ Post Workout STRETCH ☐ Post Workout WATER

Something positive from today's workout

How I feel after today's workout

MOVEMENT

Workout plan/type   Date:

Length: [ ]   Focus: [ ]

movement	reps	sets	weight	time

☐ Post Workout STRETCH   ☐ Post Workout WATER

Something positive from today's workout

How I feel after today's workout

MOVEMENT

Workout plan/Type Date:

Length: [ ] Focus: [ ]

movement	reps	sets	weight	time

☐ Post Workout STRETCH   ☐ Post Workout WATER

Something positive from today's workout

How I feel after today's workout

MOVEMENT

Workout plan/Type Date:

Length: _____ Focus: _____

movement	reps	sets	weight	time

☐ Post Workout STRETCH   ☐ Post Workout WATER

Something positive from today's workout

How I feel after today's workout

MOVEMENT

Workout plan/Type Date:

Length: [ ]   Focus: [ ]

movement	reps	sets	weight	time

☐ Post Workout STRETCH   ☐ Post Workout WATER

Something positive from today's workout

How I feel after today's workout

MOVEMENT

Workout plan/Type   Date:

Length: [ ]   Focus: [ ]

movement	reps	sets	weight	time

[ ] Post Workout STRETCH   [ ] Post Workout WATER

Something positive from today's workout

How I feel after today's workout

MOVEMENT

Workout plan/Type   Date:

Length: [ ]   Focus: [ ]

movement	reps	sets	weight	time

☐ Post Workout STRETCH   ☐ Post Workout WATER

Something positive from today's workout

How I feel after today's workout

MOVEMENT

Workout plan/type   Date:

Length: [ ]   Focus: [ ]

movement	reps	sets	weight	time

☐ Post Workout STRETCH   ☐ Post Workout WATER

Something positive from today's workout

How I feel after today's workout

MOVEMENT

Workout plan/Type   Date:

Length: [   ]   Focus: [   ]

movement	reps	sets	weight	time

☐ Post Workout STRETCH   ☐ Post Workout WATER

Something positive from today's workout

How I feel after today's workout

MOVEMENT

Workout plan/Type Date:

Length: _____ Focus: _____

movement	reps	sets	weight	time

☐ Post Workout STRETCH   ☐ Post Workout WATER

Something positive from today's workout

How I feel after today's workout

MOVEMENT

Workout plan/Type Date:

Length: [　　　] Focus: [　　　]

movement	reps	sets	weight	time

☐ Post Workout STRETCH   ☐ Post Workout WATER

Something positive from today's workout

How I feel after today's workout

MOVEMENT

Workout plan/type _____ Date: _____

Length: [   ]   Focus: [   ]

movement	reps	sets	weight	time

☐ Post Workout STRETCH   ☐ Post Workout WATER

Something positive from today's workout

How I feel after today's workout

MOVEMENT

Workout plan/Type Date:

Length: _____ Focus: _____

movement	reps	sets	weight	time

☐ Post Workout STRETCH   ☐ Post Workout WATER

Something positive from today's workout

How I feel after today's workout

MOVEMENT

Workout plan/Type   Date:

Length: [ ]   Focus: [ ]

movement	reps	sets	weight	time

☐ Post Workout STRETCH   ☐ Post Workout WATER

Something positive from today's workout

How I feel after today's workout

Nutrition

Nutrition

If you are like most women, there's a high probability that, in your lifetime, you've already experimented with diet after diet to no avail. We're regularly bombarded with marketing and advertisements of diet options that offer the promise of quick and superficial results while ditching entire food groups. Vegan, gluten-free, paleo, keto, low-carb, high fat… the buzz-words leading us to the promise of a "perfect body" are never ending. On top of that, the amount of information about which nutritional path is best for you can be daunting and overwhelming. If you have experienced this cycle of constantly wondering and testing which nutrition option is best for you, you are most definitely not alone. The thing is, there really isn't a "one-size-fits-all" approach to healthy eating. Your body will react in different ways to foods than mine, or your friends'. My body does not respond well to gluten, for example. I do not eat gluten **because my body is gluten intolerant,** not because a "gluten-free" diet promises better results.

I have not only been there myself, but have also worked with hundreds and hundreds of women who share similar experiences with trying to navigate the topic of healthy eating. I am here to share some good news: It doesn't have to be like this.

My method and approach to quality and sustainable nutrition practises is purposefully simple:

I encourage you to eat foods that are as close to their natural state as possible.

I encourage you to learn to be mindful and aware of how different foods make you feel.

Let me expand on these two points. Eating food as close to its natural state as possible is a simple practice that you can implement throughout your day, and it's incredibly straightforward. Each time you go to pick foods for your meals or snacks, simply think about whether or not this is the most natural state that the food can be in. For example, are you eating a flavoured apple nut bar, full of processed oils and added sugars, or are you having a handful of nuts and an apple? The difference between two options like these is often quite drastic when repeated consistently over time.

TIP: This does not have to be an overwhelming practice. This can just be something that you put in the back of your mind to quickly check in with when you eat throughout the day. Not every meal or snack needs to be perfect, either. Remember, choosing sustainability will be far more beneficial than trying to follow a strict deprivation diet, and will lead to greater and more long-term results every time.

The second part of my approach to nutrition has to do with becoming more aware of your body and mind when it comes to your food intake. Again, this doesn't have to be a scary and overwhelming practice. It simply means checking in with how your body feels before, during, and after eating. Through this practice, you will be able to choose supportive, nourishing foods that work with you and make you feel good, instead of making you wonder why you have heartburn or digestion issues AGAIN even though you're "eating healthy." It is important to recognize that just because a particular food is generally regarded as "healthy" doesn't mean it's a good fit for your unique body. For example, black beans are nutrient dense, but they are known to cause digestive distress in many people (bloating, gas, etc.). In addition to how your body physically feels in response to various foods, you can also start to acknowledge and recognize your emotional experiences during meals. Do certain foods evoke feelings of guilt, excitement, pleasure, fulfillment, and so on? Acknowledging these feelings and patterns can be hugely beneficial in learning what makes your body feel good!

Both of these strategies can be put to use in the following pages. Approach tracking your nutrition with excitement and curiosity. You are on an adventure to learn how to better tune into your body. It is incredible what you can learn by simply jotting down notes throughout the day. Approach this process with the goal of learning everything that you can about how your *unique body* responds to food, not with a goal of counting calories in versus calories out. There's so much more to nutrition than the amount of calories you consume.

TIP: If you've been conditioned to believe counting calories or points is "the" way to track your food, you are not alone. This was forced on us for such a long time that many women are still susceptible to thinking this is what "healthy eating" means. Instead, I challenge you to think about eating foods that don't have labels on them at all. When you count your calories, you are heavily dependent on the fact that you're reading the nutrition label to get that information. What kinds of foods don't have a nutrition label? Broccoli. Apples. Red peppers. Celery. Carrots. A high quality cut of meat or a filet of salmon. The healthiest foods are often the ones that are so natural, they don't come with labels. Food for thought!

If you focus on eating mostly natural-state foods and listening closely to your body's cues in response to food, you'll start to know exactly what kinds of foods work best for you. No matter how "healthy" you are, or how far you feel you have to go, the simple act of writing down and tracking your food intake can provide you with incredible insight into your body's nutritional preferences. If you've been eating tomatoes every day because they're a vegetable (so they must be healthy) but realize that every time you eat them you experience heartburn, you'll be armed with the autonomy to decide if you are willing to continue to give yourself heartburn in exchange for a few cherry tomatoes. This is how you start to feel more free around the topic of food; understanding how you feel and then deciding what you want to do when you know.

One very important reminder before you begin: guilt should never be a by-product of this tracker. Give yourself grace as you learn about your body, and remember that balance is an **absolute necessity** when it comes to sustainable and health-supporting nutrition.

Food is so much more than a tool to adjust our body composition (a.k.a. lose fat and tone up). Food can literally be medicine for the body. Remember, food is fuel. It's as simple as that. Choose foods that help you feel good, inside and out, and you will reap the benefits to both your physical and mental health.

NUTRITION

Water Intake: ✗ ✗ ✗ ✗ ✗ ✗ ○ ○ ○ ○   **Date:** July 29th

(scale from 1-10)

what I ate	time	environment	full/hunger	how I feel
Avocado Toast	8am	Quiet, alone	9/10	Satisfied, energized
Blackbean salad	12noon	Busy, on-the-go	5/10	Bloated, gassy
Hummus & Veg	2pm	Outside w/ friends	7/10	Ate too fast, wasn't full after lunch
Crackers & Cheese	3pm	Outside w/ friends	6/10	Felt like mindless eating, a bit guilty
Chicken, rice & broccoli	6pm	Dinner Table w/ fam	8/10	Full & fuelled
Ice Cream	6pm	Dinner Table w/ fam	6/10	Craving fulfilled, but crampy
Chips & Wine	9pm	In front of TV	8/10	Happy, a form of guilt-free self-care

Notes from today

I noticed some cramping 20 minutes after...
I really enjoyed my afternoon snacks w/ friends...
I felt really satisfied after dinner but...

NUTRITION

Water Intake ◊ ◊ ◊ ◊ ◊ ◊ ◊ ◊ ◊ ◊   Date:

what I ate	time	environment	(scale from 1-10) full/hunger	how I feel

Notes from today

NUTRITION

Water Intake ○○○○○○○○○○ Date:

what I ate	time	environment	full/hunger *(scale from 1-10)*	how I feel

Notes from today

NUTRITION

Water Intake 💧💧💧💧💧💧💧💧　　　　　　Date:

what I ate	time	environment	(scale from 1-10) full/hunger	how I feel

Notes from today

NUTRITION

Water Intake ○○○○○○○○○○ Date:

what I ate	time	environment	(scale from 1-10) full/hunger	how I feel

Notes from today

NUTRITION

NUTRITION

Water Intake 	Date:

what I ate	time	environment	(scale from 1-10) full/hunger	how I feel

Notes from today

NUTRITION

Water Intake ◊◊◊◊◊◊◊◊◊◊ Date:

what I ate	time	environment	(scale from 1-10) full/hunger	how I feel

Notes from today

NUTRITION

Water Intake Date:

what I ate	time	environment	(scale from 1-10) full/hunger	how I feel

Notes from today

NUTRITION

Water Intake ○ ○ ○ ○ ○ ○ ○ ○ ○ ○   Date:

what I ate	time	environment	(scale from 1-10) full/hunger	how I feel

Notes from today

NUTRITION

NUTRITION

Water Intake ○ ○ ○ ○ ○ ○ ○ ○ ○ ○　　　　　　　　　　Date:

what I ate	time	environment	(scale from 1-10) full/hunger	how I feel

Notes from today

NUTRITION

Water Intake ○○○○○○○○○○   Date:

what I ate	time	environment	(scale from 1-10) full/hunger	how I feel

Notes from today

NUTRITION

NUTRITION

Water Intake   Date:

what I ate	time	environment	full/hunger (scale from 1-10)	how I feel

Notes from today

NUTRITION

Water Intake ○○○○○○○○○○   Date:

what I ate	time	environment	full/hunger *(scale from 1-10)*	how I feel

Notes from today

NUTRITION

Water Intake

Date:

what I ate	time	environment	(scale from 1-10) full/hunger	how I feel

Notes from today

NUTRITION

Water Intake ◊ ◊ ◊ ◊ ◊ ◊ ◊ ◊ ◊ ◊   Date:

what I ate	time	environment	(scale from 1-10) full/hunger	how I feel

Notes from today

NUTRITION

Water Intake 　　　　　　　　　　　　　　　　　　　　Date:

what I ate	time	environment	(scale from 1-10) full/hunger	how I feel

Notes from today

NUTRITION

Water Intake ○○○○○○○○○○ Date:

what I ate	time	environment	(scale from 1-10) full/hunger	how I feel

Notes from today

NUTRITION

Water Intake 💧💧💧💧💧💧💧💧💧💧 Date:

what I ate	time	environment	full/hunger *(scale from 1-10)*	how I feel

Notes from today

NUTRITION

Water Intake ○○○○○○○○○○○   Date:

what I ate	time	environment	(scale from 1-10) full/hunger	how I feel

Notes from today

NUTRITION

Water Intake   Date:

what I ate	time	environment	full/hunger (scale from 1-10)	how I feel

Notes from today

NUTRITION

Water Intake ⬡⬡⬡⬡⬡⬡⬡⬡⬡ Date:

what I ate	time	environment	full/hunger *(scale from 1-10)*	how I feel

Notes from Today

NUTRITION

NUTRITION

Water Intake   💧 💧 💧 💧 💧 💧 💧 💧   Date:

what I ate	time	environment	full/hunger *(scale from 1-10)*	how I feel

Notes from today

NUTRITION

Water Intake ○ ○ ○ ○ ○ ○ ○ ○ ○ ○   Date:

what I ate	time	environment	full/hunger *(scale from 1-10)*	how I feel

Notes from today

NUTRITION

Water Intake 💧💧💧💧💧💧💧💧 Date:

what I ate	time	environment	full/hunger *(scale from 1-10)*	how I feel

Notes from today

NUTRITION

Water Intake ○○○○○○○○○○　　　　　Date:

what I ate	time	environment	full/hunger *(scale from 1-10)*	how I feel

Notes from today

NUTRITION

Water Intake 💧💧💧💧💧💧💧💧 Date:

what I ate	time	environment	(scale from 1-10) full/hunger	how I feel

Notes from today

NUTRITION

Water Intake 〇〇〇〇〇〇〇〇〇〇　　　Date:

what I ate	time	environment	full/hunger (scale from 1-10)	how I feel

Notes from today

NUTRITION

NUTRITION

Water Intake   Date:

what I ate	time	environment	full/hunger (scale from 1-10)	how I feel

Notes from today

NUTRITION

Water Intake ○ ○ ○ ○ ○ ○ ○ ○ ○ ○   Date:

what I ate	time	environment	full/hunger (scale from 1-10)	how I feel

Notes from today

NUTRITION

NUTRITION

Water Intake Date:

what I ate	time	environment	(scale from 1-10) full/hunger	how I feel

Notes from today

NUTRITION

Water Intake 〇〇〇〇〇〇〇〇〇〇 Date:

what I ate	time	environment	full/hunger (scale from 1-10)	how I feel

Notes from Today

NUTRITION

NUTRITION

Water Intake ◊ ◊ ◊ ◊ ◊ ◊ ◊ ◊ ◊ ◊   Date:

what I ate	time	environment	(scale from 1-10) full/hunger	how I feel

Notes from today

NUTRITION

Water Intake ○○○○○○○○○○ Date:

what I ate	time	environment	full/hunger *(scale from 1-10)*	how I feel

Notes from today

NUTRITION

Water Intake   Date:

what I ate	time	environment	(scale from 1-10) full/hunger	how I feel

Notes from today

NUTRITION

Water Intake 💧 💧 💧 💧 💧 💧 💧 💧 💧 Date:

what I ate	time	environment	(scale from 1-10) full/hunger	how I feel

Notes from today

NUTRITION

Water Intake ◊ ◊ ◊ ◊ ◊ ◊ ◊ ◊ ◊ ◊   Date:

what I ate	time	environment	(scale from 1-10) full/hunger	how I feel

Notes from today

NUTRITION

Water Intake 〇 〇 〇 〇 〇 〇 〇 〇 　　　　Date:

what I ate	time	environment	full/hunger *(scale from 1-10)*	how I feel

Notes from today

NUTRITION

Water Intake 💧 💧 💧 💧 💧 💧 💧   Date:

what I ate	time	environment	full/hunger *(scale from 1-10)*	how I feel

Notes from today

NUTRITION

Water Intake ◊ ◊ ◊ ◊ ◊ ◊ ◊ ◊ ◊ ◊   Date:

			(scale from 1-10)	
what I ate	time	environment	full/hunger	how I feel

Notes from today

NUTRITION

Water Intake ◊ ◊ ◊ ◊ ◊ ◊ ◊ ◊ ◊ ◊   Date:

what I ate	time	environment	full/hunger (scale from 1-10)	how I feel

Notes from today

NUTRITION

Water Intake ⬦⬦⬦⬦⬦⬦⬦⬦⬦⬦   Date:

what I ate	time	environment	full/hunger *(scale from 1-10)*	how I feel

Notes from today

NUTRITION

NUTRITION

Water Intake Date:

what I ate	time	environment	full/hunger *(scale from 1-10)*	how I feel

Notes from today

NUTRITION

Water Intake ⬡⬡⬡⬡⬡⬡⬡⬡⬡⬡ Date:

what I ate	time	environment	full/hunger (scale from 1-10)	how I feel

Notes from today

NUTRITION

Water Intake   Date:

what I ate	time	environment	full/hunger *(scale from 1-10)*	how I feel

Notes from today

NUTRITION

Water Intake ○○○○○○○○○○ Date:

what I ate	time	environment	full/hunger *(scale from 1-10)*	how I feel

Notes from today

NUTRITION

Water Intake   Date:

what I ate	time	environment	(scale from 1-10) full/hunger	how I feel

Notes from today

NUTRITION

Water Intake ⬦ ⬦ ⬦ ⬦ ⬦ ⬦ ⬦ ⬦ ⬦ ⬦   Date:

what I ate	time	environment	full/hunger *(scale from 1-10)*	how I feel

Notes from today

NUTRITION

Water Intake ⬦ ⬦ ⬦ ⬦ ⬦ ⬦ ⬦ ⬦ ⬦ ⬦   Date:

what I ate	time	environment	full/hunger *(scale from 1-10)*	how I feel

Notes from today

NUTRITION

Water Intake ○○○○○○○○○○ Date:

what I ate	time	environment	(scale from 1-10) full/hunger	how I feel

Notes from today

NUTRITION

Water Intake 　　　　　　　　　　　　　　　　　　　　　　　　Date:

what I ate	time	environment	(scale from 1-10) full/hunger	how I feel

Notes from today

NUTRITION

Water Intake 💧💧💧💧💧💧💧💧💧💧 Date:

what I ate	time	environment	full/hunger *(scale from 1-10)*	how I feel

Notes from today

NUTRITION

NUTRITION

Water Intake 💧💧💧💧💧💧💧💧 Date:

what I ate	time	environment	full/hunger *(scale from 1-10)*	how I feel

Notes from today

NUTRITION

Water Intake ○○○○○○○○○○○ Date:

what I ate	time	environment	(scale from 1-10) full/hunger	how I feel

Notes from today

NUTRITION

Water Intake Date:

what I ate	time	environment	full/hunger *(scale from 1-10)*	how I feel

Notes from today

NUTRITION

Water Intake ○ ○ ○ ○ ○ ○ ○ ○ ○ ○   Date:

what I ate	time	environment	(scale from 1-10) full/hunger	how I feel

Notes from today

NUTRITION

Water Intake Date:

what I ate	time	environment	(scale from 1-10) full/hunger	how I feel

Notes from today

NUTRITION

Water Intake　○ ○ ○ ○ ○ ○ ○ ○ ○ ○　　Date:

what I ate	time	environment	full/hunger (scale from 1-10)	how I feel

Notes from today

NUTRITION

Water Intake Date:

what I ate	time	environment	full/hunger *(scale from 1-10)*	how I feel

Notes from today

NUTRITION

Water Intake ⬦⬦⬦⬦⬦⬦⬦⬦⬦⬦ Date:

what I ate	time	environment	full/hunger *(scale from 1-10)*	how I feel

Notes from today

NUTRITION

Water Intake 💧💧💧💧💧💧💧💧💧💧 Date:

what I ate	time	environment	full/hunger *(scale from 1-10)*	how I feel

Notes from today

NUTRITION

Water Intake 💧💧💧💧💧💧💧💧💧💧 Date:

what I ate	time	environment	full/hunger *(scale from 1-10)*	how I feel

Notes from today

NUTRITION

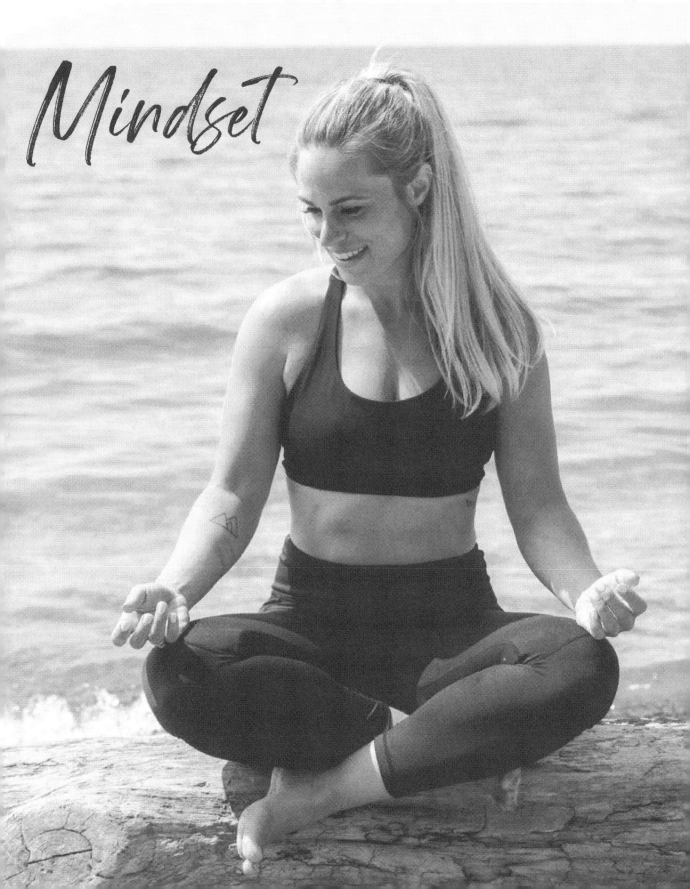

Mindset

One of the most underutilized tools when it comes to a healthy lifestyle is an awareness of — and subsequent effort to improve — **your mindset.** Study after study has proven that by practising gratitude and journaling on a regular basis, you can enhance your likelihood of accomplishing your goals. Practicing gratitude also has a direct correlation to the amount of pleasure and motivation you feel along the way.

Working on your mindset does not have to take up a lot of your time, nor does it need to be highly spiritual, "woo-woo," or far-fetched. By simply taking five minutes to fill out the following pages on a regular basis, you can not only improve the speed at which you accomplish your goals, but you will undoubtedly have more happy and positive thoughts and feelings throughout the day. Getting clear with your mindset affects your thoughts, which then affects your feelings, mood, how you handle situations and people, how you respond to things, and more. It's so important that we establish a way to get clear and steady with our minds because, as mentioned, our thoughts really can have a waterfall effect (that could potentially be negative) if you don't pay attention to managing your mindset and internal dialog. This is all about being proactive, instead of reactive.

As always, there is no pressure or "right way" to do this. Simply write down exactly what you were thinking, with no judgment to yourself, and watch your life transform as this becomes a new and enjoyable habit.

MINDSET

Date: *July 29th*

I am grateful for: *Hot coffee, my family, my health*

I am... *Thoughtful and creative. I am where I am meant to be.*

I made steps toward my goals today by...
Being kind to myself by creating a to-do list and checking off the top 3 tasks.

Something joyus/fun/positive today was...
Going on a walk with a friend

Overall Happiness Today

1 2 3 4 5 6 ⑦ 8 9 10

tommorow will be better — today was perfect

How tomorrow can be better
Taking time away from work to sit down and have lunch.

MINDSET

Date:

I am grateful for:

I am...

I made steps toward my goals today by...

Something joyus/fun/positive today was...

Overall Happiness Today

1 2 3 4 5 6 7 8 9 10

tommorow will be better   today was perfect

How Tomorrow can be better

MINDSET

Date:

I am grateful for:

I am...

I made steps toward my goals today by...

Something joyus/fun/positive today was...

Overall Happiness Today

1 2 3 4 5 6 7 8 9 10

tommorow will be better · today was perfect

How Tomorrow can be better

MINDSET

MINDSET

Date:

I am grateful for:

I am...

I made steps toward my goals today by...

Something joyus/fun/positive today was...

Overall Happiness Today

1 2 3 4 5 6 7 8 9 10

tommorow will be better   today was perfect

How Tomorrow can be better

MINDSET

Date:

I am grateful for:

I am...

I made steps toward my goals today by...

Something joyus/fun/positive today was...

Overall Happiness Today

| 1 | 2 | 3 | 4 | 5 | 6 | 7 | 8 | 9 | 10 |

tommorow will be better — today was perfect

How Tomorrow can be better

MINDSET

MINDSET

Date:

I am grateful for:

I am...

I made steps toward my goals today by...

Something joyus/fun/positive today was...

Overall Happiness Today

1 2 3 4 5 6 7 8 9 10

tommorow will be better   today was perfect

How Tomorrow can be better

MINDSET

Date:

I am grateful for:

I am...

I made steps toward my goals today by...

Something joyus/fun/positive today was...

Overall Happiness Today

1   2   3   4   5   6   7   8   9   10

tommorow will be better							today was perfect

How Tomorrow can be better

MINDSET

MINDSET

Date:

I am grateful for:

I am...

I made steps toward my goals today by...

Something joyus/fun/positive today was...

Overall Happiness Today

1 2 3 4 5 6 7 8 9 10

tommorow will be better   today was perfect

How tomorrow can be better

MINDSET

Date:

I am grateful for:

I am...

I made steps toward my goals today by...

Something joyus/fun/positive today was...

Overall Happiness Today

1   2   3   4   5   6   7   8   9   10

tommorow will be better   today was perfect

How tomorrow can be better

MINDSET

MINDSET

Date:

I am grateful for:

I am...

I made steps toward my goals today by...

Something joyus/fun/positive today was...

Overall Happiness Today

1   2   3   4   5   6   7   8   9   10

tommorow will be better   today was perfect

How tomorrow can be better

MINDSET

Date:

I am grateful for:

I am...

I made steps toward my goals today by...

Something joyus/fun/positive today was...

Overall Happiness Today

1 2 3 4 5 6 7 8 9 10

tommorow will be better today was perfect

How tomorrow can be better

MINDSET

MINDSET

Date:

I am grateful for:

I am...

I made steps toward my goals today by...

Something joyus/fun/positive today was...

Overall Happiness Today

1 2 3 4 5 6 7 8 9 10

tommorow will be better   today was perfect

How Tomorrow can be better

MINDSET

Date:

I am grateful for:

I am...

I made steps toward my goals today by...

Something joyus/fun/positive today was...

Overall Happiness Today

| 1 | 2 | 3 | 4 | 5 | 6 | 7 | 8 | 9 | 10 |

tommorow will be better																	today was perfect

How tomorrow can be better

MINDSET

MINDSET

Date:

I am grateful for:

I am...

I made steps toward my goals today by...

Something joyus/fun/positive today was...

Overall Happiness Today

1 2 3 4 5 6 7 8 9 10

tommorow will be bettertoday was perfect

How tomorrow can be better

MINDSET

Date:

I am grateful for:

I am...

I made steps toward my goals today by...

Something joyus/fun/positive today was...

Overall Happiness Today

1 2 3 4 5 6 7 8 9 10

tommorow will be better   today was perfect

How tomorrow can be better

MINDSET

Date:

I am grateful for:

I am...

I made steps toward my goals today by...

Something joyus/fun/positive today was...

Overall Happiness Today

1   2   3   4   5   6   7   8   9   10

tommorow will be better   today was perfect

How tomorrow can be better

MINDSET

Date:

I am grateful for:

I am...

I made steps toward my goals today by...

Something joyus/fun/positive today was...

Overall Happiness Today

1 2 3 4 5 6 7 8 9 10

tommorow will be better　　　　　　　　　　　today was perfect

How tomorrow can be better

MINDSET

MINDSET

Date:

I am grateful for:

I am...

I made steps toward my goals today by...

Something joyus/fun/positive today was...

Overall Happiness Today

1   2   3   4   5   6   7   8   9   10

tommorow will be better   today was perfect

How Tomorrow can be better

MINDSET

Date:

I am grateful for:

I am...

I made steps toward my goals today by...

Something joyus/fun/positive today was...

Overall Happiness Today

1   2   3   4   5   6   7   8   9   10

tommorow will be better   today was perfect

How tomorrow can be better

MINDSET

MINDSET

Date:

I am grateful for:

I am...

I made steps toward my goals today by...

Something joyus/fun/positive today was...

Overall Happiness Today

1   2   3   4   5   6   7   8   9   10

tommorow will be better   today was perfect

How Tomorrow can be better

MINDSET

Date:

I am grateful for:

I am...

I made steps toward my goals today by...

Something joyus/fun/positive today was...

Overall Happiness Today

1   2   3   4   5   6   7   8   9   10

tommorow will be better   today was perfect

How Tomorrow can be better

MINDSET

MINDSET

Date:

I am grateful for:

I am...

I made steps toward my goals today by...

Something joyus/fun/positive today was...

Overall Happiness Today

1 2 3 4 5 6 7 8 9 10

tommorow will be better   today was perfect

How tomorrow can be better

MINDSET

Date:

I am grateful for:

I am...

I made steps toward my goals today by...

Something joyus/fun/positive today was...

Overall Happiness Today

| 1 | 2 | 3 | 4 | 5 | 6 | 7 | 8 | 9 | 10 |

tommorow will be better — today was perfect

How Tomorrow can be better

MINDSET

MINDSET

Date:

I am grateful for:

I am...

I made steps toward my goals today by...

Something joyus/fun/positive today was...

Overall Happiness Today

1   2   3   4   5   6   7   8   9   10

tommorow will be better   today was perfect

How tomorrow can be better

MINDSET

Date:

I am grateful for:

I am...

I made steps toward my goals today by...

Something joyus/fun/positive today was...

Overall Happiness Today

1 2 3 4 5 6 7 8 9 10

tommorow will be better

today was perfect

How tomorrow can be better

MINDSET

MINDSET

Date:

I am grateful for:

I am...

I made steps toward my goals today by...

Something joyus/fun/positive today was...

Overall Happiness Today

1 2 3 4 5 6 7 8 9 10

tommorow will be better   today was perfect

How tomorrow can be better

MINDSET

Date:

I am grateful for:

I am...

I made steps toward my goals today by...

Something joyus/fun/positive today was...

Overall Happiness Today

1   2   3   4   5   6   7   8   9   10

tommorow will be better					today was perfect

How Tomorrow can be better

MINDSET

MINDSET

Date:

I am grateful for:

I am...

I made steps toward my goals today by...

Something joyus/fun/positive today was...

Overall Happiness Today

1 2 3 4 5 6 7 8 9 10

tommorow will be better   today was perfect

How tomorrow can be better

MINDSET

Date:

I am grateful for:

I am...

I made steps toward my goals today by...

Something joyus/fun/positive today was...

Overall Happiness Today

1 2 3 4 5 6 7 8 9 10

tommorow will be better   today was perfect

How Tomorrow can be better

MINDSET

Date:

I am grateful for:

I am…

I made steps toward my goals today by…

Something joyus/fun/positive today was…

Overall Happiness Today

1 2 3 4 5 6 7 8 9 10

tommorow will be better *today was perfect*

How tomorrow can be better

MINDSET

Date:

I am grateful for:

I am...

I made steps toward my goals today by...

Something joyus/fun/positive today was...

Overall Happiness Today

1   2   3   4   5   6   7   8   9   10

tommorow will be better   today was perfect

How Tomorrow can be better

MINDSET

MINDSET

Date:

I am grateful for:

I am…

I made steps toward my goals today by…

Something joyus/fun/positive today was…

Overall Happiness Today

1   2   3   4   5   6   7   8   9   10

tommorow will be better   today was perfect

How tomorrow can be better

MINDSET

Date:

I am grateful for:

I am...

I made steps toward my goals today by...

Something joyus/fun/positive today was...

Overall Happiness Today

1 2 3 4 5 6 7 8 9 10

tommorow will be better   today was perfect

How Tomorrow can be better

MINDSET

MINDSET

Date:

I am grateful for:

I am...

I made steps toward my goals today by...

Something joyus/fun/positive today was...

Overall Happiness Today

1 2 3 4 5 6 7 8 9 10

tommorow will be better   today was perfect

How tomorrow can be better

MINDSET

Date:

I am grateful for:

I am...

I made steps toward my goals today by...

Something joyus/fun/positive today was...

Overall Happiness Today

1   2   3   4   5   6   7   8   9   10

tommorow will be better　　　　　　　　　　　today was perfect

How Tomorrow can be better

MINDSET

MINDSET

Date:

I am grateful for:

I am...

I made steps toward my goals today by...

Something joyus/fun/positive today was...

Overall Happiness Today

1　2　3　4　5　6　7　8　9　10

tommorow will be better today was perfect

How tomorrow can be better

MINDSET

Date:

I am grateful for:

I am...

I made steps toward my goals today by...

Something joyus/fun/positive today was...

Overall Happiness Today

| 1 | 2 | 3 | 4 | 5 | 6 | 7 | 8 | 9 | 10 |

tommorow will be better — today was perfect

How Tomorrow can be better

MINDSET

MINDSET

Date:

I am grateful for:

I am...

I made steps toward my goals today by...

Something joyus/fun/positive today was...

Overall Happiness Today

1   2   3   4   5   6   7   8   9   10

tommorow will be better   today was perfect

How tomorrow can be better

MINDSET

Date:

I am grateful for:

I am...

I made steps toward my goals today by...

Something joyus/fun/positive today was...

Overall Happiness Today

1   2   3   4   5   6   7   8   9   10

tommorow will be better   today was perfect

How Tomorrow can be better

MINDSET

Date:

I am grateful for:

I am...

I made steps toward my goals today by...

Something joyus/fun/positive today was...

Overall Happiness Today

1   2   3   4   5   6   7   8   9   10

tommorow will be better   today was perfect

How tomorrow can be better

MINDSET

Date:

I am grateful for:

I am...

I made steps toward my goals today by...

Something joyus/fun/positive today was...

Overall Happiness Today

1 2 3 4 5 6 7 8 9 10

tommorow will be better — today was perfect

How tomorrow can be better

MINDSET

MINDSET

Date:

I am grateful for:

I am...

I made steps toward my goals today by...

Something joyus/fun/positive today was...

Overall Happiness Today

1   2   3   4   5   6   7   8   9   10

tommorow will be better   today was perfect

How tomorrow can be better

MINDSET

Date:

I am grateful for:

I am...

I made steps toward my goals today by...

Something joyus/fun/positive today was...

Overall Happiness Today

1 2 3 4 5 6 7 8 9 10

tommorow will be better — today was perfect

How Tomorrow can be better

MINDSET

MINDSET

Date:

I am grateful for:

I am...

I made steps toward my goals today by...

Something joyus/fun/positive today was...

Overall Happiness Today

1   2   3   4   5   6   7   8   9   10

tommorow will be better   today was perfect

How tomorrow can be better

MINDSET

Date:

I am grateful for:

I am...

I made steps toward my goals today by...

Something joyus/fun/positive today was...

Overall Happiness Today

1 2 3 4 5 6 7 8 9 10

tommorow will be better   today was perfect

How Tomorrow can be better

MINDSET

MINDSET

Date:

I am grateful for:

I am...

I made steps toward my goals today by...

Something joyus/fun/positive today was...

Overall Happiness Today

1 2 3 4 5 6 7 8 9 10

tommorow will be better   today was perfect

How Tomorrow can be better

MINDSET

Date:

I am grateful for:

I am...

I made steps toward my goals today by...

Something joyus/fun/positive today was...

Overall Happiness Today

1   2   3   4   5   6   7   8   9   10

tommorow will be better   today was perfect

How Tomorrow can be better

MINDSET

Date:

I am grateful for:

I am...

I made steps toward my goals today by...

Something joyus/fun/positive today was...

Overall Happiness Today

1   2   3   4   5   6   7   8   9   10

tommorow will be better   today was perfect

How Tomorrow can be better

MINDSET

Date:

I am grateful for:

I am…

I made steps toward my goals today by…

Something joyus/fun/positive today was…

Overall Happiness Today

1 2 3 4 5 6 7 8 9 10

tommorow will be better · today was perfect

How tomorrow can be better

MINDSET

MINDSET

Date:

I am grateful for:

I am...

I made steps toward my goals today by...

Something joyus/fun/positive today was...

Overall Happiness Today

1   2   3   4   5   6   7   8   9   10

tommorow will be better   today was perfect

How tomorrow can be better

MINDSET

Date:

I am grateful for:

I am...

I made steps toward my goals today by...

Something joyus/fun/positive today was...

Overall Happiness Today

1   2   3   4   5   6   7   8   9   10

tommorow will be better   today was perfect

How Tomorrow can be better

MINDSET

MINDSET

Date:

I am grateful for:

I am…

I made steps toward my goals today by…

Something joyus/fun/positive today was…

Overall Happiness Today

1 2 3 4 5 6 7 8 9 10

tommorow will be better — today was perfect

How tomorrow can be better

MINDSET

Date:

I am grateful for:

I am...

I made steps toward my goals today by...

Something joyus/fun/positive today was...

Overall Happiness Today

1   2   3   4   5   6   7   8   9   10

tommorow will be better   today was perfect

How Tomorrow can be better

MINDSET

MINDSET

Date:

I am grateful for:

I am...

I made steps toward my goals today by...

Something joyus/fun/positive today was...

Overall Happiness Today

1   2   3   4   5   6   7   8   9   10

tommorow will be better   *today was perfect*

How tomorrow can be better

MINDSET

Date:

I am grateful for:

I am…

I made steps toward my goals today by…

Something joyus/fun/positive today was…

Overall Happiness Today

| 1 | 2 | 3 | 4 | 5 | 6 | 7 | 8 | 9 | 10 |

tommorow will be better   today was perfect

How Tomorrow can be better

MINDSET

MINDSET

Date:

I am grateful for:

I am...

I made steps toward my goals today by...

Something joyus/fun/positive today was...

Overall Happiness Today

1 2 3 4 5 6 7 8 9 10

tommorow will be better   today was perfect

How Tomorrow can be better

MINDSET

Date:

I am grateful for:

I am...

I made steps toward my goals today by...

Something joyus/fun/positive today was...

Overall Happiness Today

1   2   3   4   5   6   7   8   9   10

tommorow will be better   today was perfect

How tomorrow can be better

MINDSET

MINDSET

Date:

I am grateful for:

I am...

I made steps toward my goals today by...

Something joyus/fun/positive today was...

Overall Happiness Today

1 2 3 4 5 6 7 8 9 10

tommorow will be better   today was perfect

How Tomorrow can be better

MINDSET

Date:

I am grateful for:

I am...

I made steps toward my goals today by...

Something joyus/fun/positive today was...

Overall Happiness Today

1   2   3   4   5   6   7   8   9   10

tommorow will be better   today was perfect

How Tomorrow can be better

MINDSET

MINDSET

Date:

I am grateful for:

I am...

I made steps toward my goals today by...

Something joyus/fun/positive today was...

Overall Happiness Today

1 2 3 4 5 6 7 8 9 10

tommorow will be better   today was perfect

How Tomorrow can be better

MINDSET

Date:

I am grateful for:

I am...

I made steps toward my goals today by...

Something joyus/fun/positive today was...

Overall Happiness Today

1 2 3 4 5 6 7 8 9 10

tommorow will be better	today was perfect

How tomorrow can be better

MINDSET

About the Author

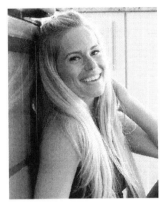

Jeenie Brasseur is the founder and CEO of KeepFit Women, a Canadian wellness company that helps women reach their whole-body fitness and health goals with sustainable programs and coaching. Jeenie has an honours Bachelor of Arts in Recreation Therapy and a diploma in Social Work Studies. She is a Certified Personal Trainer, a certified Nutrition and Weight Management coach, a Pre and Postnatal Exercise Specialist, and a certified Level 2 Reiki Practitioner. As a sought-after Fitness Coach and Mentor, she has become obsessed with helping women feel strong, fit, confident, and supported through KeepFit Women's award winning movement and nutrition programs, and inside her inclusive KeepFit Women Community.

Jeenie is a mom of three and is married to her best friend, Steve. She enjoys spending quality time with her family, creating quick and easy recipes, working out in her garage gym, enjoying good wine with friends, and sharing her fitness journey on her social media platforms.

FOR FREEBIES AND OTHER BONUS RESOURCES, SCAN THE CODE!

www.keepfitwomen.com/keepfittracker

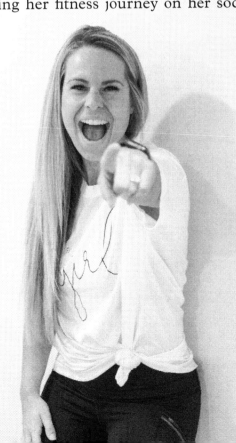

Manufactured by Amazon.ca
Bolton, ON